SOME HERBS THAT CAN KEEP YOU HEALTHY

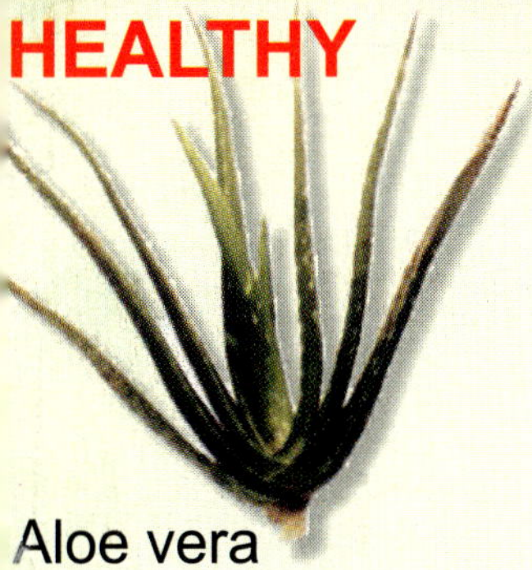

Aloe vera
is an amazing
wound healer.

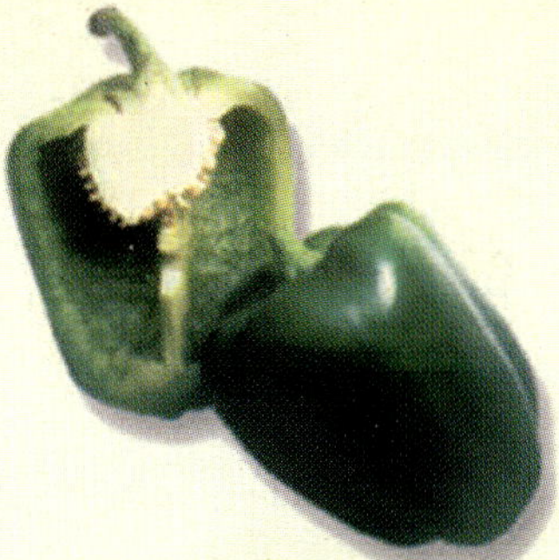

Green peppers
have anti inflammatory
properties.

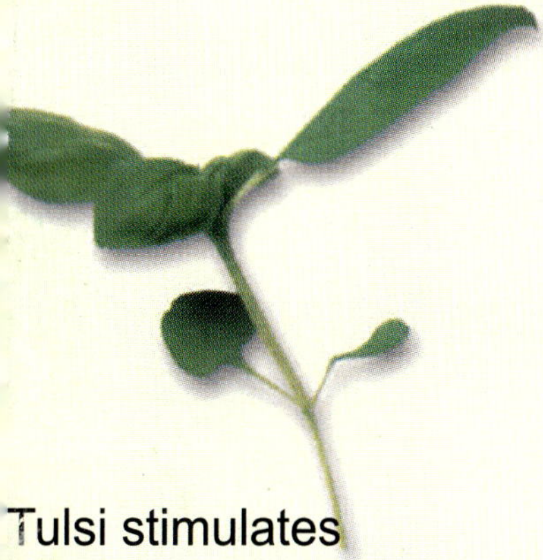

Tulsi stimulates
the immune system
and improves digestion.

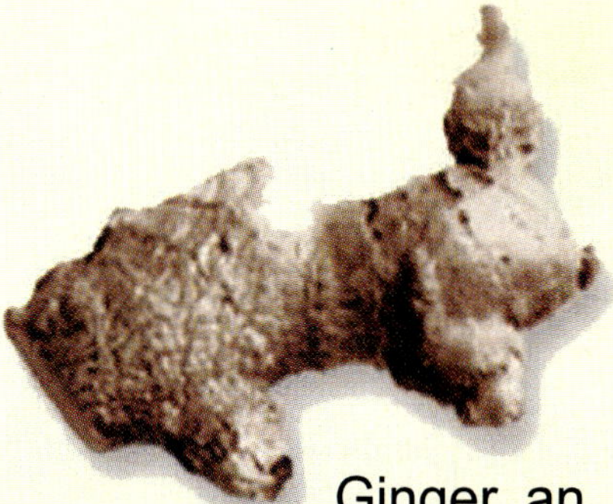

Ginger, an
expectorant, aids
digestion, too.

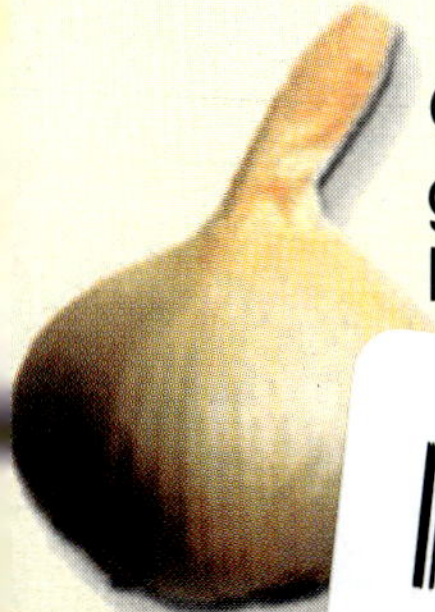

Garlic is a
great immunity
booster.

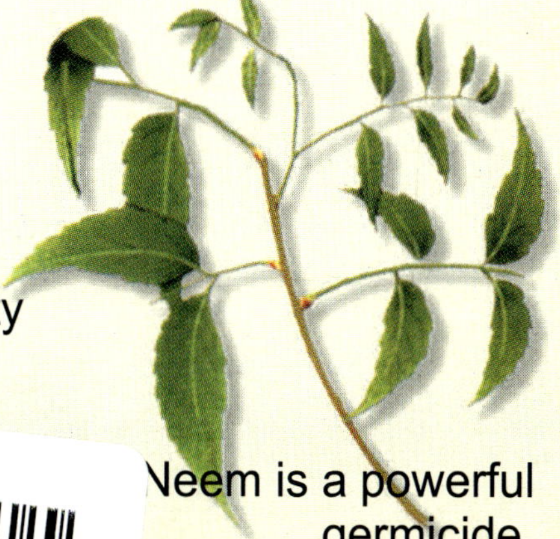

Neem is a powerful
germicide.

Memory Concentration *naturally*

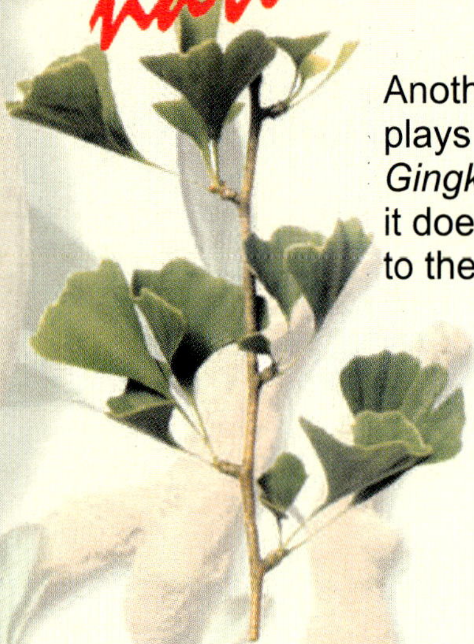

Another valuable herb that plays a role in enhancing memory is *Gingko biloba* — it does so by improving circulation to the brain.

Herbal remedies with Brahmi can benefit young and old alike.

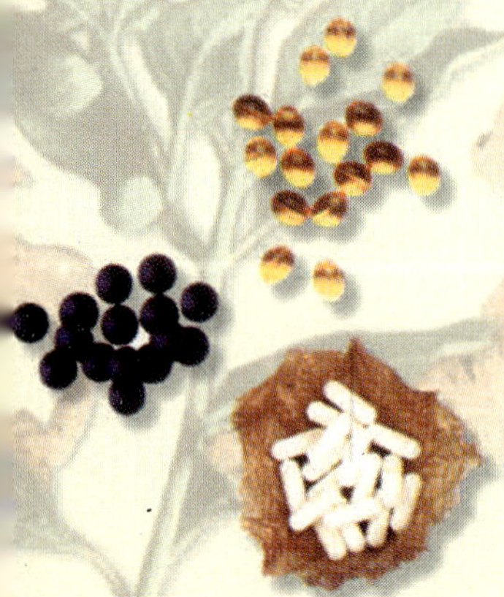

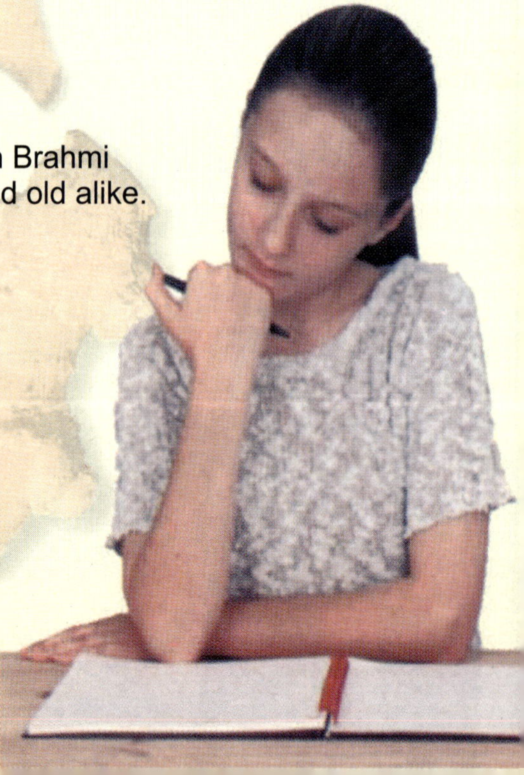

How to improve and

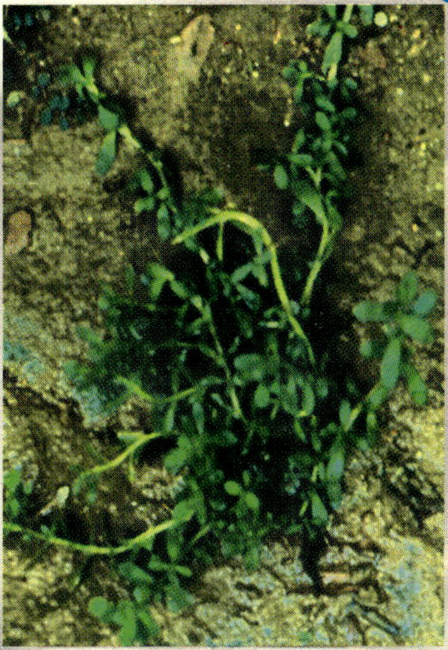

Brahmi stimulates the nervous system, thereby improving mental function, memory and concentration and reducing learning time.

Scientists stress a diet rich in vitamins B^1, B^6, B^{12} and C; as well as choline, folate, niacin, calcium, copper, iodine, iron, magnesium, manganese, potassium, zinc and, above all, lecithin.

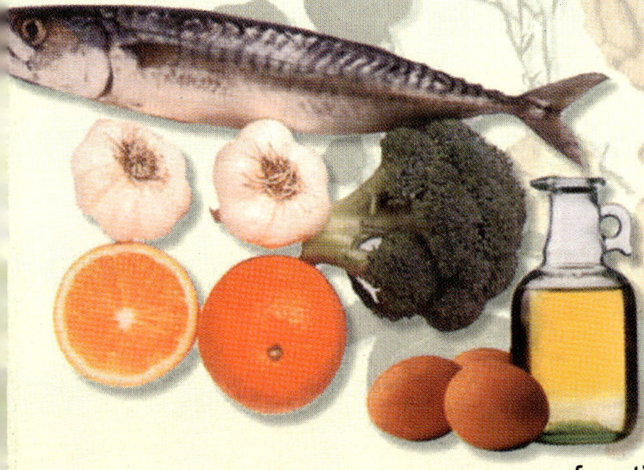

Eggs and sunflower oil contain lecithin, which enhances functioning of the brain.

Experts are now examining the power of certain herbs that sharpen memory.

In some people brain cells degenerate with ageing at 40 — in others the memory may be razor-sharp even at 80.

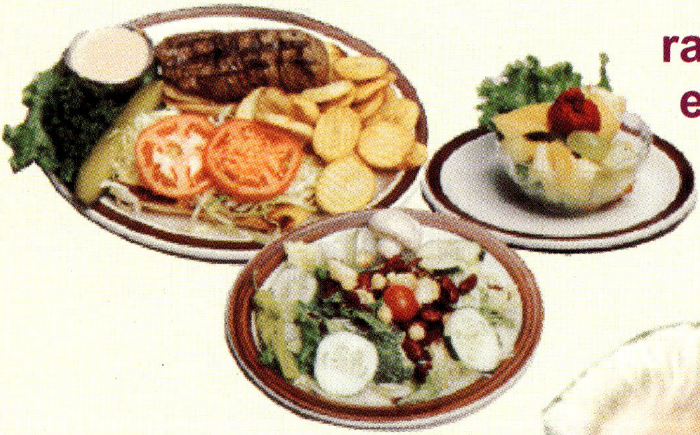

EAT HEALTHY,
STAY HEALTHY

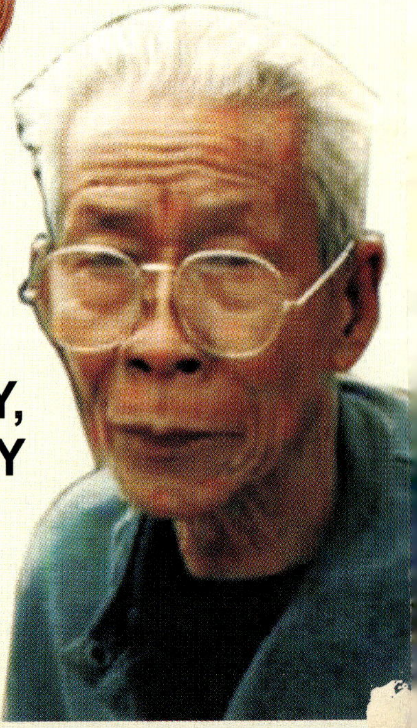

The natural way to health 1

Discover the amazing power of herbs

Brahmi

(Bacopa monnieri)

The Brain Tonic

Brijesh Regal

UNICORN BOOKS Pvt. Ltd.

Distributors

PUSTAK MAHAL

UNICORN

Publishers
UNICORN BOOKS Pvt. Ltd. New Delhi-110002

Distributors
Pustak Mahal, Delhi-110006

Sales Centres
• 6686, Khari Baoli, Delhi-110006, *Ph:* 3944314, 3911979
• 10-B, Netaji Subhash Marg, Daryaganj, New Delhi-110002,
Ph: 3268292, 3268293, 3279900 • *Fax:* 011-3280567

Administrative Office
J-3/16 (Opp. Happy School), Daryaganj, New Delhi-110002
Ph: 3276539, 3272783, 3272784 • *Fax:* 011-3260518
E-mail: unicornbooks@vsnl.com • *Website:* www.pustakmahal.com

Branch Offices

BANGALORE: 22/2, Mission Road (Shama Rao's Compound), Bangalore-560027, *Ph:* 2234025 • *Fax:* 080-2240209 *E-mail*: rapidexblr@satyam.net.in

MUMBAI: 23-25, Zaoba Wadi (Opp. VIP Showroom), Thakurdwar, Mumbai-400002, *Ph:* 2010941 • *Fax:* 022-2053387 *E-mail*: rapidex@bom5.vsnl.net.in

PATNA: Khemka House, 1st Floor (Opp. Women's Hospital), Ashok Rajpath, Patna-800004, *Telefax:* 0612-673644

HYDERABAD: 5-1-707/1, Brij Bhawan, Bank Street, Koti, Hyderabad-500095, *Ph:* 4737530 • *Fax:* 040-4737290

ISBN.: 81-780-6041-8

Warning and Disclaimer: While every care has been taken to ensure that only validated information has been presented, the author, editor and publishers have neither the liability nor responsibility for any loss or damage that may be caused, directly or indirectly, by the information contained in this book. It is recommended that a physician be consulted before taking any herbal remedy.

Edition : 2002

Printed at : Param Offsetters, Okhla, New Delhi-20

Acknowledgements

The Editor gratefully acknowledges the contributions and guidance provided by Sanat Products Limited and the Dabur Research Foundation in the preparation of this booklet.

The design and artworks for this booklet were prepared by the RAKA Associates creative team.

Other Books

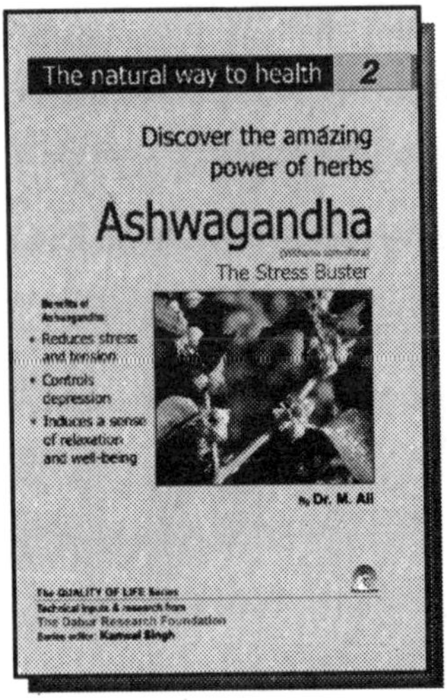

The natural way to health 2
Discover the amazing power of herbs
Ashwagandha
The Stress Buster
Reduces stress and tension
Controls depression
Induces a sense of relaxation and well-being
By Dr. M. Ali
The QUALITY OF LIFE Series
The Dabur Research Foundation

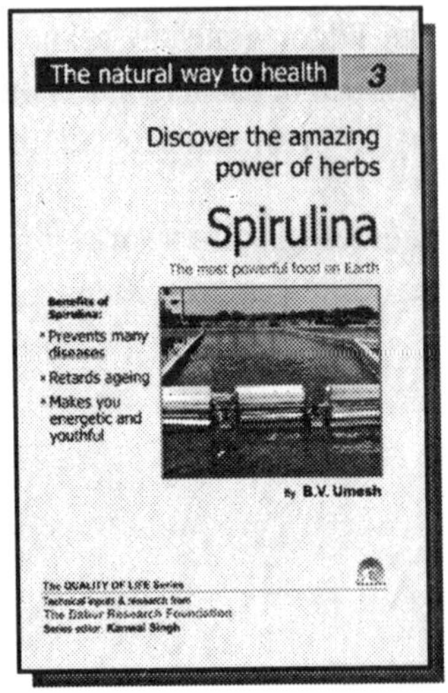

The natural way to health 3
Discover the amazing power of herbs
Spirulina
The most powerful food on Earth
Benefits of Spirulina:
Prevents many diseases
Retards ageing
Makes you energetic and youthful
By B.V. Umesh
The QUALITY OF LIFE Series
The Dabur Research Foundation
Series editor: Kanwal Singh

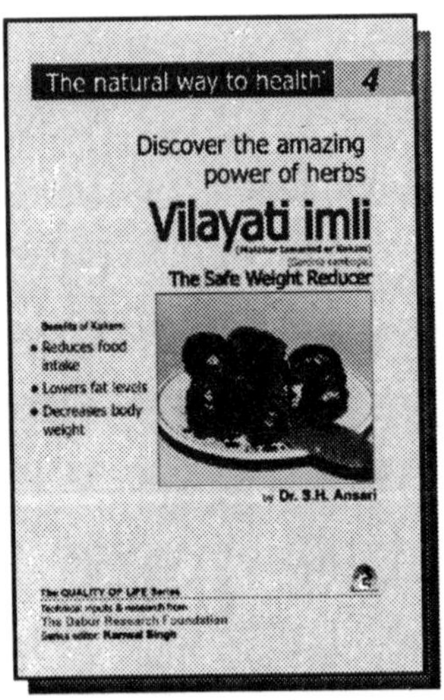

The natural way to health 4
Discover the amazing power of herbs
Vilayati imli
The Safe Weight Reducer
Reduces food intake
Lowers fat levels
Decreases body weight
By Dr. S.H. Ansari
The QUALITY OF LIFE Series
The Dabur Research Foundation
Series editor: Kanwal Singh

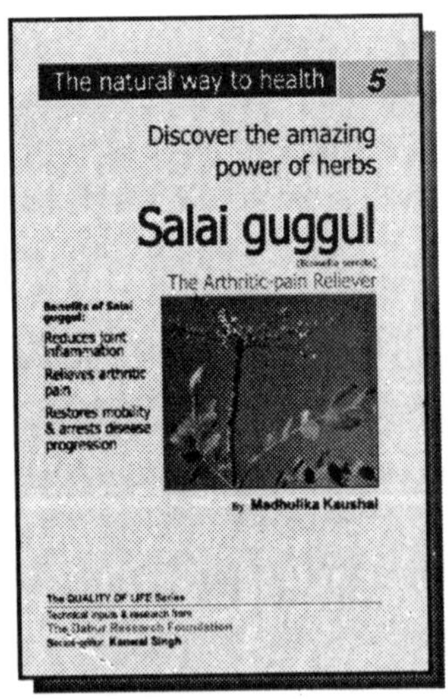

The natural way to health 5
Discover the amazing power of herbs
Salai guggul
The Arthritic-pain Reliever
Reduces joint inflammation
Relieves arthritic pain
Restores mobility & arrests disease progression
By Madhulika Kaushal
The QUALITY OF LIFE Series
The Dabur Research Foundation
Series editor: Kanwal Singh

Preface

As head of the Dabur Research Foundation, I have, for many years, been excited by the remarkable potential of herbs for promoting health and well-being. Certainly, this will come as no surprise to those of you who are familiar with, or have trusted, traditional Ayurvedic remedies for preventing and treating health disorders. What might surprise you, however, is that modern clinical studies and trials have now scientifically endorsed the therapeutic properties of many common and not-so-common herbs, and that such remedies are increasingly becoming popular with Western medical practitioners. One of the reasons for the resurgence of traditional herbal remedies is their proven efficacy combined with safety.

I was, therefore, delighted to learn that a series of simply written booklets is planned to spread awareness about the multiple health benefits of many indigenously available plants. At last, many more people will know why the world has recognised the usefulness of nutraceuticals for treating and preventing a host of common ailments, and chronic disorders – like arthritis, obesity, nutritional deficiencies, stress, memory loss, constipation, and the like.

It is my hope that readers will, henceforth, evaluate the natural options available to them for their own ailments. There is no doubt in my mind that they will greatly benefit from the remarkable properties of herbal remedies.

—D.B.A. Narayana
Dabur Research Foundation

The super-computer that is the human mind

The human mind is truly an amazingly complex and efficient process house.

Even in this age of super-computers, the human mind towers above them all. We have all read about people such as the chess grandmasters (like Gary Kasparov) who can defeat computers, of maths wizards (such as Shakuntala Devi) who can solve complex questions faster than any machine, and of scientists who can invent formulae no computer ever could.

Remarkable feats of memory are a part of Indian tradition. We know that the *Vedas* were orally transmitted for centuries before they were written down. According to Mr A.K. Ramanujam in *Uncollected Poems and Prose*, the techniques for memorising them included not only grammatical and phonetic analyses, but various pedagogic methods of marking each uttered phrase physically by various gestures and bodily movements—so that the texts were inscribed almost into the body's motor memory.

Mr Ramanujam cites meeting an 80-year-old Vedic scholar who could, without a moment's pause, repeat any part of the *Rig Veda* from any point to any point, backwards, omitting every other line, give you a concordance of any word or phrase you chose, citing its use throughout the entire text, and so on!

Some remarkable modern feats of memory

There are mindboggling reports about people who can simultaneously do several activities, displaying remarkable skills of mind and memory.

How many of us could, for instance, emulate the skill displayed by a Jain monk who could do eight things simultaneously: repeat without change a poem that was recited to him by one person, answer several questions from philosophy, arithmetic and the local newspaper put to him by three other persons, play a game of dice with another person, play a game of chess with yet another, complete a half-finished verse recited by a seventh person, and accurately give the count of the number of pebbles being thrown all the while on his bare back!

Most of us do not need the level of memory skills narrated above to lead normal lives. Yet, there are many among us who face embarrassing moments when our memory fails us and we wish there was something we could do to remedy it. Now, experts tell us, we can.

But first, it is important to ascertain the causes of a failing memory or weakened concentration.

Does this sound familiar?

Do you belong to that group of people who are forever searching for names, belongings, details... as depicted in this poem?

Just a line to say I'm living;
That I'm not among the dead;
That I'm getting more forgetful,
And more mixed up in the head.

For, sometimes I can't remember,
When I stand at the foot of the stair,
If I must go up for something,
Or I've just come down from there.

And, before the fridge, so often,
My mind is filled with doubt
Have I just put the food away,
Or, have I come to take some out?

And, there are times when it's dark out,
With my night cap on my head,
I don't know if I'm retiring,
Or have just got out of bed.

So, if it's my turn to write you,
There is no need to get sore.
I may think I may have written,
And don't want to be a bore.

Remember, I do love you,
And I wish that you were here
But it's nearly mail time,
So I must say, "Goodbye, dear."

There I stood beside the mailbox,
With a face so very red,
Instead of mailing you my letter,
I had opened it instead!

—Amir C. Tuteja

What is your memory problem?

All people suffer from minor memory lapses, but serious memory loss should not be neglected.

There is none among us who can not be accused of occasional memory lapses... that important letter that did not get written... that birthday that was forgotten... that familiar face that haunts you... mixing up the date of the exam... missing the train or losing your keys...

Different people suffer from different kinds of memory disorders. There are people who have problems with short-term habitual memory, such as forgetting to turn off the alarm clock in the morning, or locking the car. There are people with long-term episodic memory problems. They may forget to pass on messages, for instance. And, finally, there could be problems with internally cued memory, such as with people who forget the reason why they entered a room or why they picked up a phone. A total or partial loss of memory is known as amnesia.

Sure, it happens occasionally to every person. It only becomes worrying when it happens too often, or at too young an age. If you see yourself in the character portrayed in the poem on the previous page, then it is time to take stock and find out what is aggravating the memory lapses and what, if anything, you could be doing about it.

The findings of latest research

After 40, for most of us, there is a marked slowdown in our reaction times, our concentration span and powers of memory...

A recent article by Mike Collett-White, distributed by Reuters, presented latest research on memory conducted by Keith Wesnes, honorary professor of psychology at Northumbria University. The professor says research proves that reaction times, concentration span and powers of memory start to decline markedly from the age of 40-45 onwards.

His conclusions are based on a study of nearly 2,300 healthy people aged between 18 and 87. While the ability to retain information and recognise words, pictures and digits did not decrease significantly until well into the 60s, the slowdown in speed at which people could "drag up" the information came much sooner. "By the time you reach middle age you can be 10 to 15 per cent slower to react than when you are in your 20s," says Wesnes.

While the exact reasons for the slowdown in carrying out cognitive tasks have not been established, they may be related to the efficiency of the brain's transmitter system. *"The efficiency of this transmitter system decreases in our 40s and 50s,"* explains James Semple, a brain specialist at Addenbrookes Hospital in Cambridge.

Common causes of memory lapses

Memory loss could be temporary or permanent. If brain cells that facilitate memory are damaged, they cannot be healed.

The reason for a sudden loss of concentration or forgetfulness could be simply an outcome of undue tension or anxiety. However, it can cause some individuals to show physical symptoms of illness; they may even begin to demonstrate psychosomatic illnesses – and memory impairment.

Nutritional deficiencies or malnutrition are also known to impair brain cells and damage memory. The Intelligence Quotient (IQ) of undernourished children is often way below those with proper and adequate nourishment.

Memory loss could be temporary or permanent, as in amnesia. This could be the result of an injury, accident or trauma. Sometimes, the tissue surrounding the injury compensates and the memory is partially restored. Sometimes, the brain cells that facilitate memory are permanently damaged. Since brain cells cannot heal themselves or regenerate, the memory loss may be permanent or serious.

Still another cause is degeneration of brain cell tissues due to the ageing process. In some people, this may take place at around 40 years or so, in others the memory may be razor-sharp even into their 80s. There is no norm.

Poor nourishment can affect the memory

Proper nutrition is absolutely essential, especially before birth and during childhood.

Scientists have found a relationship between nutrients and the brain's ability to learn and remember. According to them, a lack of certain nutrients can lead to memory and other cognitive failures. The maximum damage is caused to the foetus if it does not receive adequate nourishment in the mother's womb. Nutritionists also recommend that infants are breastfed in order to give them a sound start. Thereafter, the first few years of a child are the most critical. Medical science has proven that the younger you are, the more easily you can learn and remember. Therefore, nourishing food is important during the school years.

Scientists stress a diet rich in the following nutrients, all of which seem related to memory: vitamins B1 (thiamine), B6, B12, and C, choline, folate, niacin, calcium, copper, iodine, iron, magnesium, manganese, potassium, zinc, and – above all – lecithin.

Proper nutrition also means staying away from certain harmful substances. Alcohol consumption and tobacco use, for instance, are known to hasten ageing and impair the memory. Young people drinking three to four units of alcohol effectively slow down their reaction times to those of someone who is 60 or over.

Choose the memory aid that works for you

Do not despair! Memory can be sharpened and common forms of forgetfulness are curable. Use the memory aid that works best for you.

There are some people who never forget a telephone number or a birth date, and never have to consult their address books. There are others with a photographic memory for words – never forgetting a spelling once they have seen it in print. Still other persons never forget a face and may always be able to link the right name to the right face.

While some of the above talents may be natural abilities that people are born with, many others claim that, with the right discipline, the brain can be trained to sharpen cognitive ability. There are no formulae, unfortunately, for building an iron-clad memory – what works for one person may not work for another.

For example, some persons create acronyms to help them remember a long list. Others cannot remember the acronym in the first place! They may have to use other devices that suit them, like creating word associations or links. Needless to say, they could end up making hilarious mistakes! An elderly person reminded herself when she was introduced to a stranger that she would never forget his name because she would associate it with a mass of water falling. So she smiled confidently when she waved goodbye, saying cheerily, "Bye, Mr Waterfall!" He was not amused for his name was Fountain!

Simple techniques to an improved memory

Different memory aids work for different people. Some popular techniques are enumerated here. Read on to find out what works best for you.

The acronym approach: Suppose you have to memorise the names of six cities: Agra, Etawah, Lucknow, Gwalior, Bangalore and Nagpur. To start with, take the first alphabets A, E, L, G, B, N and create a new word from them: This word could be BANGLE. Then, just remember that one word to help you trigger all the names with each letter of the alphabet.

Jot down, make lists: Another successful method is to write down important facts, and list all the things to do. Writing will reinforce the recall, because you read and write and see the words on the list.

Aural-visual images: Take a visual mind-picture of where you place something important; then say it out aloud. This will give an aural and visual image, and help you remember it when you need it.

Read a lot: It helps to sharpen the memory, so read. Some people find reading aloud helps.

Some more common aids to the memory

The methods listed here have been found to work for other people. You can create your own special ways of remembering.

There are so many spy novels that tell of special agents memorising coded information and then throwing away the paper on which it was written. Have you ever wondered how they did it? Well, here are some more ways for you:

Cues: Tie a ribbon on a finger; put on the alarm; look for prominent markers or cues; they will all trigger the name of the action you need to take, the place you must visit, or whatever.

Chunking: Think how you remember a phone number or a longish credit-card number. Take this number for example: 970573204545. You could break it up into convenient chunks instead of remembering each numeral, thus 9705 7320 4545. It becomes easier that way.

Word-associations or links: Make meaningful associations that will act as a memory trigger. Here's how someone learnt to remember a new phone number: 916389583. First, he broke it up into convenient chunks, thus: 916 38 95 83. 916 was the area exchange, so that was not difficult to remember. 38 was his car number so he could remember that. The last two digits, 83 were the reverse of the first two digits. And 95 was his grandmother's age — and that went in between. And he had memorised it all!

The 'use it or lose it' theory

A healthy lifestyle can slow down the degenerative process. Take regular physical exercise and keep the brain stimulated.

Regular exercise keeps the body and the mind invigorated. It increases the supply of blood and, hence, oxygen to the lungs, the brain and the heart and keeps you healthy. A healthy lifestyle can certainly slow down the degenerative processes. But when modern-day specialists talk about exercise, they do not mean physical exercise alone.

The latest theory, featured on a popular television programme recently, was the "Use it or lose it theory", also advocated by the brain specialist, Dr Semple, in the Reuters' article quoted earlier in this booklet. Quite simply, it means that the brain functions better and longer, the more people exercise their brain. Stop using it and it begins to rust, so to speak. Therefore, keep the brain cells challenged and stimulated by regular mental exercise. Staying mentally active will keep the memory alert and sharpen it over time.

And, lastly, you can depend on natural herbs to prevent anxiety and to keep your memory in good fettle – one such herb is **Brahmi** (*Bacopa monnieri*), best recommended for its preventive and restorative powers.

What the *National Geographic* and the *Discovery Channel* say

A prestigious magazine and a television channel suggest it's time to keep an open mind about time-tested and clinically validated herbal remedies.

In the early part of the year 2000, the *National Geographic* magazine took a closer look at alternative herbal remedies from around the world. Among the herbs featured was *Saw palmetto* and *Centella asiatica*, or Mandookaparni – a close cousin of the indigenous **Brahmi** or *Bacopa monnieri.* The long, colourfully illustrated feature reflects the growing interest of the world community in alternative treatments.

Discovery Channel, too, has shown a rekindled interest in alternative and complementary treatments through its regular weekly programmes in which alternative therapies are exhaustively scrutinised and presented.

Some 20 years ago, we had scarcely heard of the powers of Reiki, or Pranic healing, or Kerala Ayurveda. Today, people are turning to gem therapy, aromatherapy and yoga as easily as they once turned to homoeopathy as the only alternative to allopathy.

The power of natural herbs should be easier to comprehend. After all, the animal kingdom has always relied on nature for all its cures. As have tribal people from all around the world. As did our grandmothers, in their days. All of us will remember the soothing power of *mulethi* with honey for that sore throat; the efficacy of *laung* in treating that persistent toothache; the application of *haldi* in hot oil for covering a wound.

What the experts say about herbs for memory loss

Many renowned scientists believe in the healing powers of herbs, particularly for slowing down ageing and consequent memory loss.

What should interest us, however, is that according to Dr Wesnes, honorary professor of psychology at Northumbria University, herbal medicine was a possible way of staving off the effects of ageing on memory.

Dr Wesnes quotes a study in which a concoction made from the herb, *Gingko biloba*, was used for an extended period by 256 middle-aged people. The results: it improved memory by over seven per cent, although it did not improve the speed. The effect was sustained some two weeks after the cessation of dosing.

In Chinese herbalism, herbs to aid memory include fleeceflower root and black ginger seed. The Chinese treat memory loss caused by stress or fatigue with Chinese wolfberry. In the science of herbalism, they may recommend ginseng powder to act as a memory aid or stimulant; or they may suggest you add gotu kola to your food and drink for several days to revive your memory. Rosemary and sage are also considered useful in refreshing the memory.

Studies conducted with *Bacopa monnieri* or **Brahmi** have demonstrated encouraging results, too. These are cited towards the latter part of this booklet. Needless to say, the importance of essential nutrients in the diet, especially B vitamins and protein for amino acids, are necessary for the brain to function efficiently. Eggs and sunflower oil contain lecithin, which also enhances brain functioning.

Now, discover the power of herbs for yourself

There is a herb out there for every ailment. Many cultures and tribes still rely on the therapeutic properties of common herbs. So can you.

Open your mind, and discover the wonderful world of nutraceuticals – remedies made from the roots, stems, leaves and flowers of common or not-so-common plants, trees, shrubs – all classified as herbs.

Choose from herbs for a wide variety of ailments: there are food supplements out there full of unbelievable nutrients; there are miraculous remedies for relieving the agony of arthritis and restoring mobility; there are herbal supplements that can help you slim, or restore stamina or relieve stress and fatigue.

Those of us who are fortunate enough to live in the Himalayas can find a treasure trove of herbs as we wander through the forests and valleys, and make our own decoctions, infusions or teas, poultices and extracts. Others, who live in the cities, can turn to practising *ayurvaids* for their needs or buy commercial brands.

This booklet tells you about the amazing properties of **Brahmi** and where you can source remedies based on it.

About Brahmi and where it can be found

Brahmi is a well-known indigenous herb that grows abundantly in the warm, temperate and tropical climates of South Asia.

A man was showing off his garden in the Guntur region of Andhra Pradesh to a friend when suddenly she stooped down and plucked the stem of a herb with several roundish leaves. Why, she said excitedly, you have **Brahmi** growing wild in your garden. Did you know my grandmother used to grind some **Brahmi** leaves with soaked, crushed almonds and insist we eat them every morning on waking up when I was a school girl? She said it would help us in our schoolwork. The woman nibbled at the leaf and gave it to her friend to do the same. The taste was slightly bitter.

If you read about **Brahmi**, you will discover that it grows abundantly in warm, moist, temperate and tropical climates, especially in Southern Asia. In India, it is found in marshy places of the North and South at altitudes of around 1,300m. It can also be cultivated easily in damp areas and propagated by seed and also vegetatively.

See for yourself what the plant looks like in the centrespread of this booklet. You may not know it but you may have the very answer to your memory problems growing right in your backyard!

Why Brahmi should be the herb of choice

Brahmi improves mental function, but is prescribed for a host of other conditions too.

The entire plant — the root, the stalk and the leaves — constitutes the well-known formulation we call **Brahmi**. The herb is an astringent, cooling, bitter, stimulating and moistening and is widely used in various remedies. It improves mental function, memory and concentration and reduces learning time. It is used in the indigenous system of medicine for the treatment of asthma, hoarseness, insanity, epilepsy and as a potent nervine tonic, cardiotonic and diuretic. In China, it is also taken as a tonic for impotence, premature ejaculation, infertility and rheumatic conditions.

Brahmi acts, principally, by stimulating the central nervous system. It aids in the elimination of fluids, shrinks tissues, decreases fatigue and depression, which also impacts 'memory-ability'. Hence, **Brahmi** is recommended not just for improved concentration and memory functions, but also for rheumatism, blood disease, mental disorders, high blood pressure, sore throat, tonsillitis, cystitis, and stress, among other conditions.

Brahmi is used in many Ayurvedic preparations

The herb forms an important ingredient of a number of Ayurvedic preparations such as Brahmighritam, Brahmirasayan, etc.

In traditional uses, **Brahmi** leaves are used as a diuretic, and an aperient in cases of snake bite. The juice of the leaves is given to children for relief in bronchitis and diarrhoea. The powder of leaves is used in treating asthenia and nervous breakdowns. Powdered leaves, with some black pepper, are used in setting bone fractures. Leaf juice with petroleum is effective as a remedy for rheumatism.

Leaves mixed with clarified butter are used to treat hoarseness, as a brain tonic, in treatment of anxious neurosis, nervous weakness and to sharpen dull memory.

The plant is also useful in vitiated conditions, biliousness, neuralgia, inflammations, splenomegaly, ascites, flatulence, leucoderma, dysmenorrhoea, elephantiasis and general debility.

But it is the effect of **Brahmi** on learning ability that most interests us in this booklet.

Special constituents of Brahmi

The herb, Brahmi, contains many compounds that are useful in treating a host of health problems.

The herb, **Brahmi**, contains alkaloids, saponins, sterols, sugar, and minerals apart from other constituents such as D-mannitol, betulic acid, heptacosane, octacosane, nonacosane, etc., that are present in smaller quantities.

Other compounds available in the herb are Bacosides A, and A3, hersaponin, betulic acid, monnierin, alkaloid herpestine and brahmine, flavonoids leutcolin, 7 glucosides and apigenin.

They can be quantified by the application of modern techniques, such as HPLC and HPTLC.

How should one take Brahmi?

All parts of the Brahmi herb are beneficial — the leaves, stem, roots are all used to make potions, oils, creams, infusions.

Formulations of **Brahmi** can be safely consumed as a beverage in moderate dosages, as a capsule, or used as a compress and massage oil, a poultice, tea and skin cream.

Brahmi infusion, when taken as a beverage, can improve circulation in the legs and treat varicose veins. In some cases, it can also act as a soporific in treating insomnia.

But it is as a nerve tonic that it is most effective. It is recommended especially for young students, for professionals who want to keep their memories sharp and for older persons who fear the onset of memory loss.

It is best to buy standardised formulations commercially available from a reputed manufacturer, as it is not possible to prepare an equally effective memory-enhancing tonic at home.

Here's how you can make an infusion with Brahmi:

Pour 2 cups of boiling water over 1 teaspoon of the herb. Let it steep for 10 minutes. Drink up to 2 cups a day, adding lemon or honey for taste, if desired.

Clinical validation of Brahmi in animals - 1

Research has demonstrated the efficacy of Brahmi in strengthening the memory in many animal studies.

Effect on learning ability

The synergistic effect of *Bacopa monnieri and Centella asiatica* was tested on the learning ability of albino mice. The albino mice were intubated with the extract of both for 120 days and demonstrated a significant improvement in their learning behaviour.*

Effect on avoidance learning during endurance performance

A nine-week, cross-over study [5 weeks of a polyherbal preparation administration with 4 weeks withdrawal] was performed on albino rats. Results indicated a significant improvement in avoidance learning during endurance performance due to the intake of the drug containing *Bacopa monnieri, Withania somnifera, Celastrus paniculatus, Centella asiatica* and *Evolvulus alsinoides.* ^

---

*Ambuganapathi, B., *International Seminar on Recent Trends in Pharmaceutical Sciences*, Ootacamund, Feb. 1995.

^Bharadwaj S.K.; Srivastava K.K.; *Indian J. of Exp. Biol,* 33, 1995.

Clinical validation of Brahmi in animals - 2

Brahmi is a herb with apparent anti-anxiety and memory-strengthening characteristics, as several more animal studies have demonstrated.

Learning performance

In one study, conducted to ascertain its effect on learning performance, it was found that the **Brahmi**-treated group exhibited better acquisition, improved retention and delayed extinction. In an active conditioned flight, the drug-treated animals showed a shorter reaction time than the control group. In a continuous avoidance group also, the drug-administered group showed better performance than the control group.*

In another study, *Bacopa monnieri* (**Brahmi**) in crystalline form was administered once a day between 9.00 am and 10.00 am. Electric shock was used as the aversive experience and the latency to step down from a raised wooden platform was the behavioural measure. Memory of the aversive experience in the control group was found to be less at the age of 15 and 21 months than what it was at the age of three and nine months. **Brahmi** offset this loss and led to improvement in the memory at the geriatric levels (15 and 21 months).*

---

*Gupta, B.S.; Gupta, U.; S.P. Dubey, G.P., *International Seminar on Free Radicals Mediated Diseases & Ayurveda,* Faculty of Ayurveda, IMS, BHU, Varanasi, India, Sept. 1996.

Clinical validation of Brahmi in humans - 1

Human studies have also reinforced the remarkable memory-enhancing properties of Brahmi.

Memory-enhancing effect in human studies

A herbal preparation containing *Bacopa monnieri* (**Brahmi**), *Acorus calamus, Piper longum, Valeriana wallichii, Rauwolfia serpentina, Conium maculatum* and *Vitis vinifera* was given for 110 to 117 days at the dose of 500 mg (2 tabs of 250 mg each) a day to all the students. An overall freshness and improvement in daily routine without fatigue was observed in all the students. An improved memory and concentration was also observed.[#]

The synergistic effect of *Bacopa monnieri* and *Centella asiatica* was studied on school children. The students administered with *Bacopa monnieri* and *Centella asiatica* syrup showed a marked improvement in their examination performance. No side-effects were observed during and after the study.*

The effect of a micro-medicine derived from *Bacopa monnieri* over a 9-month treatment on 110 boy students with average intelligence, in the age range of 10-13 years was studied. Mean differences in post-testing and pre-testing IQ scores in the experimental group were statistically significant as compared to the control group.[$]

#Suru, P.A.; Sardeshmukh, S.P., *Ayurved Research Papers II, 1995.*

*Ambuganapathi, B., *International Seminar on Recent Trends in Pharmaceutical Sciences*, Ootacamund, Feb. 1995.

$Abhang, R., *J. of Res. in Ayur. and Siddha*, 1993.

Other benefits of Brahmi

Brahmi is found to be effective in relieving mental fatigue, improving mental function, managing heart disease and inhibiting cancer.

Management of heart disease

A formulation made of *Bacopa monnieri, Inula racemosa* and *Commiphora mukul* showed good results in the management of ischaemic heart disease.*

Anti-cancer activity (in-vitro study)

The alcoholic plant extract of *Bacopa monnieri* has been reported to have anti-cancer properties. Different concentrations of ethanol extract of the plant were tested with sarcoma-180 cell culture. All the essential parameters like cell growth, viability and 3H-thymidine incorporation into the DNA were evaluated. The extract-treated cases showed that the sarcoma-180 cell growth was significantly inhibited with increasing concentrations of *Bacopa monnieri*. Hence, the alcoholic extract of **Brahmi** can be considered as an anti-cancer drug.**

---

*Sharma, S.D.; Upadhyay, B.N.; Tripathi, S.N., *J. Natl. Integ. Med. Assoc.,* 26 (9), 249-53, 1984.

**Elangovan, V; Govindaswamy, S; Rammorthy, N.; Balakrishna, K. *Fitoterapia* v. 67(3): p. 274, 1996.

How Brahmi has helped some people

"I can't remember when I last forgot!"

—Meera Asnani, Jaipur

"It was always so embarrassing. I would meet someone — the face would be familiar, but the name would evade me. Things got to a head when I forgot where I placed my valuables — jewellery, my passport, my cheque book and the like. Then, there were problems with my concentration.

"I consulted a physician. He told me this was to be expected at my age. Me, old? At 52? I was depressed for a few days. Finally, I consulted a well-known herbalist. He prescribed a herbal remedy consisting of small spatula-shaped leaves and told me to take them with clarified butter for a few months. He told me the leaves were from an indigenous, creeping, succulent herb called Brahmi.

"The difference was amazing. Within a few months, I felt my memory sharpening. I felt less anxious about problems that had seemed insurmountable in the past, and my confidence returned. My herbalist was as pleased as I was with the results. But then, we got transferred away from the city and I panicked. Where would I be able to obtain the Brahmi *leaves? No problem, said the herbalist. You can buy herbal remedies containing extract of* Brahmi *from chemists, and he gave me several brand names.*

"My poor memory is now a thing of the past. I am approaching 60 now, and never forget the things I should remember. Especially, I never forget to take my Brahmi *capsules regularly."**

---

*From an unsolicited letter written to Sanat Products Limited, Delhi.

A student narrates his experience with Brahmi

"I no longer fear examinations!"

—Rajesh Mittal, Agra

"Examination time was a great ordeal for me. I would become tense days before an impending exam. As the time got nearer, I would suffer from sleeplessness, anxiety and the fear of failure. My concentration would be affected. I would take hours memorising simple facts. My appetite would also be affected, as well as my digestion. The morning of the exam, I would wake up puking and suffer from loose motions. My condition would affect the whole household.

"Then my grandmother came to stay. The exams were yet a few months away, but already, the strain was beginning to tell. Dadi took matters into her own hands. 'He is not eating right,' she announced to my mother's dismay. 'But, Maaji, I give him balanced meals and supplement it with vitamins,' Mother protested. 'Where can you find me Brahmi *leaves?' asked Dadi, firmly. We asked around, without much success. Ask a* vaid, *we were advised.*

"Well, that was the end of our search. And, soon, the end of my problem. Within a few weeks of taking Brahmi *as prescribed, I felt my concentration sharpening. Learning became fun as I never forgot a lesson, even after one reading. I no longer suffered from a bad case of nerves before the test. And my results were gratifying.*

"My father says it was a placebo effect. I don't care. Thank you, Brahmi!"*

---

*An unsolicited testimonial sourced from Dabur Research Foundation, Delhi.

Are all herbs safe and efficacious?

Like with any food or drink, prudent use of herbs is recommended. Although they are natural, they must not be taken in excess.

Think of a herb as you think of any other nutritious plant vegetable — carrots, lettuce, beans, cauliflower, onions, ginger.... Do you worry about consuming them? No, because you know that they are unlikely to have undesirable side-effects.

Of course, all vegetables don't agree with everybody. Some people may get indigestion with a particular food, others may get acidity; so it is with any medicinal herb. If you should feel any discomfort after taking any herbal remedy, stop taking it and consult your herbalist or doctor.

Remember, if you want to be sure that you are getting a standardised extract or remedy, then turn to the brands offered by various reputed nutraceutical companies. The well-known among them invest in cultivating their own herbs and extracting the oils through scientific techniques, and they monitor the output to ensure that what you get is consistent quality. They will also share the findings of the latest clinical trials with their customers — including which side-effects to expect. They will also prescribe the right dosage.

Look up their websites for detailed information.

For more information

For all those interested in knowing more about this amazing herb, there are many printed reports.

Effect of Bacopa monnieri linn (Brahmi) on avoidance responses in rats

Singh H.K. et al. (1982), J. of Ethnopharmacology, 5, 205-214.

Studies on the anti-anxiety effect of the Medhya Rasayana Drug, Brahmi (B. monnieri)

Singh R.H. et al. (1979), Jour. Res. Ind. Med. Yoga & Homeo 14:3-6

Indian Herbal Pharmacopoeia Vol.I

Compendium of Indian Medicinal Plants

Rastogi R.P. & Mehrotra B.N., Vol.I pg. 53, Vol. II pg. 91, Vol. III pg. 88, Vol. IV pg. 96.

Indian Herbal Remedies

Khare C.P., pg. 121-123

Study to evaluate the effect of micro (Suksma) medicine derived from Brahmi on students of average intelligence

Abhang R., (1992), J.R. AS., Vol. XIV, No. 1-2, pg. 10-24